Forgotten Home Apothecary

Discover Potent Remedies for
Everyday Ailments

ISBN 978-1-300-81062-9
Noah Heath
Copyright@2024

TABLE OF CONTENT

CHAPTER 1 3
   INTRODUCTION 3
CHAPTER 2 8
   Setting Up Your Home Apothecary 8
CHAPTER 3 14
   Harvesting and Preparing Ingredients 14
CHAPTER 4 20
   Creating Herbal Remedies 20
CHAPTER 5 27
   Remedies for Common Ailments 27
THE END 57

CHAPTER 1

INTRODUCTION

How do you make a home apothecary? What it means and how it fits into history

A home apothecary is like a personal pharmacy where you can make and store natural medicines. The word apothecary comes from the time when apothecaries were the first pharmacists and made and sold plant medicines, mixtures, and treatments. These professionals were very good at herbalism. They used their understanding of plants and natural substances to heal and treat a wide range of illnesses.

In the past, every home had some kind of home pharmacy, which was usually run by the family mother. There were dried herbs, potions, poultices, and other natural medicines that had been passed down from generation to generation in these apothecaries. Before the development of modern medicine and drugs, it was very important to know what plants to use and how to prepare them. Home apothecaries have been around for a long time and represent a close relationship with nature and a self-sufficient approach to health and wellness.

Relevance and Resurgence of Interest in the Modern World

A growing desire for natural and organic health solutions has led to a big rise in interest in home apothecaries over the past few years. This movement fits in with a larger movement toward sustainability, healthy living, and going back to more traditional ways of doing things in many areas of life.

The modern home apothecary shows that people are becoming more aware of how useful natural medicines can be. More and more people are learning about the problems that could happen if they only use manufactured drugs, like the side effects and damage to the environment. Also, people are becoming more and more appreciative of how simple, pure, and effective natural medicines are.

The resurgence is also helped by how easy it is to get knowledge. People can now easily learn how to recognize, grow, harvest, and use medicinal plants thanks to the many websites, books, and online communities that are committed to herbalism and natural remedies. Making knowledge more accessible to everyone has given many people the confidence to start their own home pharmacies.

Natural remedies have many benefits.
Good for your health

Natural medicines are good for your health in many ways, and they can often treat a wide range of common illnesses in a gentle and effective way. When compared to many traditional drugs, they tend to be less invasive and have fewer side effects. It's good for your health in these ways:

Holistic Healing: Natural remedies often treat the reasons of health problems instead of just making the symptoms better. Taking a more whole-person approach can lead to health changes that last longer.

Boosts Immunity: Many herbs and natural ingredients, like garlic, echinacea, and elderberry, are known to support and boost the immune system. This helps keep you healthy and avoid getting sick.

Reduces Inflammation: Turmeric, ginger, and chamomile are some of the strong anti-inflammatory ingredients that can help with arthritis, digestive problems, and chronic pain.

Herbal remedies like St. John's wort, lavender, and valerian root are often used to treat stress, anxiety, and sadness, which is good for both mental and emotional health.

Effects on the Environment

Other things that are good for the environment are using natural medicines and keeping a home apothecary. How to do it:

Chemical Use Is Cut Down: When people choose natural remedies instead of synthetic ones, they use fewer chemicals that are bad for the earth during the manufacturing process.

Sustainable Sourcing: Many natural remedies can be gathered in a sustainable way from home gardening or legal wild harvesting, which lowers the carbon footprint of making and transporting commercial drugs.

Less Waste: Natural remedies often come in containers that can be used again and again, like glass jars and bottles, instead of the single-use plastic packaging that is popular in the drug industry. This helps make less trash and smog.

Benefits for the economy

A home apothecary is good for your health and the world, and it can also help your wallet in big ways:

Cost-effective: It can be much cheaper to grow your own herbs and make your own medicines than to buy over-the-counter medicines. Once you've set up your home apothecary, the only things that will cost you regularly are seeds, dirt, and maybe some new containers.

Self-Sufficiency: Having an apothecary at home makes you more independent and less reliant on public health care services. This can be especially helpful when money is tight or when there aren't many healthcare options available.

Support the local economy: When you buy veggies and other things you can't grow or find yourself, shopping at local farmers' markets can help the local economy grow and keep your money in the area.

CHAPTER 2

Setting Up Your Home Apothecary

Important Equipment and Tools
Bottles, jars, and other containers

A good range of jars, bottles, and other containers is an important part of any home apothecary. These are important for keeping your home treatments fresh and effective for as long as possible when you store them. You'll need the following key types:

You can store dried herbs and bulk items in glass jars. Pick jars that don't let air in to keep your veggies fresh.

Amber bottles are great for saving tinctures, infused oils, and other mixtures that don't like light. Amber glass keeps things safe from UV light, which can make medicines less effective.

Spray bottles are useful for making and using plant sprays for things like bug sprays and room sprays.

Salve Tins: You can store creams and salves in small tins. They are easy to carry and store.

Dropper bottles are necessary for accurately giving tinctures and liquid medicines.

Mason Jars: Mason jars are easy to find and can be used to store and make soups, decoctions, and even fermentations.

Using Scales and Tools to Measure

When you make your own medicines, accuracy is very important to make sure they work and are safe. So, it is necessary to have the right measure tools.

Digital Scale: A digital scale lets you measure weight instead of volume, which is often a more accurate way to do it. When working with strong herbs and essential oils, this is especially important for accuracy.

Cups and measuring spoons: For recipes that call for specific amounts of items by volume, you need a set of measuring spoons and cups that you can trust.

Graduated Cylinders and Beakers: These are great for measuring liquids and let you make exact amounts of ingredients.

A pestle and mortar

One of the first tools used in plant medicine was a mortar and pestle. This important tool is used to grind and crush herbs to get their healing effects out. This is why it's important:

Flexibility: You can use it to turn dried herbs into fine powders or to crush fresh herbs to get the oils out of them.

Control: If you grind the herbs by hand, you can change the consistency and coarseness, which is useful for some recipes.

Tradition: Using a mortar and pestle brings you closer to the old ways of herbalism, which makes the craft more enjoyable and meaningful.

Basic Things You Need to Stock Up on Common Herbs and What They Do

It is important to have a number of common herbs in your home apothecary so that you can treat a wide range of illnesses. Here are some important plants and what they're used for:

Chamomile: Chamomile is known to be calming, and it can be used to make teas that help with sleeplessness, stress, and anxiety. It can also reduce inflammation, which makes it useful in skin care products.

Lavender is a useful herb that is often used to calm people down. It can help you relax and sleep by adding it to drinks, tinctures, and baths. Lavender oil is also often used in aromatherapy and on the skin to treat small cuts and stings.

Peppermint: Peppermint is great for stomach problems. Its leaves can be made into a tea that can help with headaches, sickness, and indigestion. The essential oil can be put on the skin to ease pain or used in aromatherapy.

Echinacea: This vegetable is known to help the immune system. It can be used to make teas and medicines that treat and stop colds and the flu.

Calendula: The leaves of the calendula plant are known to help heal skin. You can mix them with oils to make balms and salves that are good for cuts, burns, and rashes.

Ginger: Ginger, whether it's fresh or dried, is often used to help people who feel sick and make digestion better. It can also be used in drinks and tinctures and is known to help with inflammation.

Oils of essential

Essential oils are highly concentrated plant products that have the smell and health benefits of the plant. Here are some important essential oils that you should have in your house pharmacy:

A lot of people use lavender essential oil to calm down and rest. When softened, it can be put on the skin, added to baths, or used in diffusers.

Tea Tree Oil: This oil is known to kill germs and fungi. You can use it to heal skin problems like pimples, athlete's foot, and cuts.

Peppermint Oil: When applied topically (diluted), it can help with headaches and muscle pain. Its energizing smell can also be used in aromatherapy.

Eucalyptus oil is great for breathing problems. It can be steamed and breathed in to clear out the lungs and ease coughs.

Rosemary Oil: This oil is known to be exciting and can help you focus and remember things better. It can also be used to make hair grow faster.

Butter and base oils

Butters and base oils are used to carry essential oils and herbs so that they can be safely put on the skin. In addition, they are good for you in their own ways.

Coconut oil is a multipurpose oil that can kill germs and keep skin moist. It can be used to make lotions, salves, and creams.

Olive Oil: Olive oil is great for infusions and as a base for salves and ointments because it is full of vitamins and healthy fats.

Jojoba Oil is a liquid wax that is very similar to sebum, which is the skin's natural oil. It works great for hair products and serums for the face.

Shea Butter: It keeps skin soft and smooth and is full of vitamins A and E. You can use it to make body butters and lip balms.

Chocolate Butter: Because it is rich and softening, cocoa butter is great for making thick creams and lotions that are great for dry skin.

CHAPTER 3

Harvesting and Preparing Ingredients

Getting Herbs to Grow
The best plants to grow at home

It's fun and useful to grow your own herbs because they give you a steady supply of ingredients for your home pharmacy. Here are some good herbs to start with:

Basil: Basil is used in cooking, but it can also be used as medicine because it can reduce inflammation and kill germs.

Mint: Peppermint and spearmint are great for stomach problems and make teas and tinctures taste cool.

Lavender: This flower has a lovely scent and can help you relax. It can be used in aromatherapy, teas, and salves.

Rosemary: This strong plant is great for improving memory and focus, and it's also easy to grow.

Thyme is a strong antiseptic plant that can be used to make tea that can help with coughs and sore throats.

Chamomile: Chamomile is an important flower for teas and skin treatments because it calms people down.

A hardy plant that does well in most areas is echinacea, which is often used to boost the immune system.

How to Plant Herbs and Take Care of Them

You don't need to have a green thumb to grow herbs at home, but here are some basic tips to make sure your plants stay healthy and produce lots of herbs:

Pick the Right Spot: Most herbs do best in a sunny area that gets at least six hours of sunshine a day. To grow herbs indoors, put them near a window that faces south or use grow lights.

Quality of the Soil: Use organically rich soil that drains well. Soil that is too wet will kill herbs, so make sure it drains well.

When you water herbs, be careful not to give them too much water. It's best to keep the dirt damp, not wet.

Space: Allow enough room for each flower to grow. Plants are more likely to get diseases when there is less air flow because of too many people around them.

Harvesting: Trim your flowers often to make them grow bushier. Pick the plants in the morning, after the dew has dried but before it gets too hot for the oils to stay fresh.

Protection against pests: To keep your veggies bug-free, use natural ways to protect them, like neem oil or neighbouring plants.

Looking for Food in the Wild
How to Find and Gather Wild Herbs

Looking for herbs in the wild can be a fun way to add new items to your home pharmacy. But you need to know about it and be careful:

Research and Identification: Use field books, apps, or foraging groups to learn about local plants that can be eaten or used for medicine. Get used to how plants look at different times of the year.

Start with Safe Herbs: Start with herbs that are easy to spot, like dandelion, nettle, and plantain, which are known for their uses and don't look much like other plants.

How to pick: Only take what you need when you pick and leave enough for the plant to keep growing. To keep the plant from getting hurt, use clean, sharp tools.

Ethical Ways to Go Foraging

Ethical foraging makes sure that wild plants can keep growing and be used by future generations:

Follow the rule of thirds when harvesting: take only a third of what's there, leaving plenty for the plant and other animals that eat plants.

Respecting Nature: Don't bother animals or hurt the environment. Follow well-worn routes and foraging spots.

Legal Things to Think About: Make sure that hunting is legal where you are going. On some public and private areas, you are not allowed to pick plants.

How to Dry and Store Herbs
Different Ways to Dry Herbs

To keep herbs' strength and stop mold growth, they must be dried correctly:

For air drying, tuck small groups of herbs together and hang them upside down in a warm, dry place with good air flow.

Herbs that don't have much water in them, like thyme, rosemary, and oregano, work well with this method.

Dehydrator: A food dehydrator lets you dry herbs quickly and evenly in a controlled setting. Set the temperature to about 35°C (95°F) and check it often.

If you don't have a dehydrator, you can dry things in the oven by setting it to the lowest temperature. On a baking sheet, spread out the herbs. Leave the oven door slightly open to let the steam escape. Keep a close eye on things to avoid burning.

Microwave Drying: You can use a microwave for small amounts. Put the herbs between two pieces of paper towel and dry them in the microwave for 30 seconds at a time on low power. Be careful with this method because the herbs can easily get too hot.

How to Store Things Correctly

If you store dried herbs the right way, they will keep their health benefits and taste for longer:

Containers: To keep dried herbs safe from air, wetness, and light, store them in containers that don't let air in. It works best in glass jars with caps that fit tightly.

Labeling: Write the name of the herb and the date it was dried on the lid of every jar. This helps you keep track of how fresh they are.

Place to store: Keep your plant containers somewhere cool and dark. Herbs can lose their quality if they are exposed to light, heat, or wetness.

Shelf Life: Dried herbs usually stay strong for about a year. After that, they might lose some of their medicinal and flavorful benefits.

CHAPTER 4

Creating Herbal Remedies

Basic Recipes for Infusions and Teas to Treat Common Illnesses

Some of the easiest and most powerful ways to use herbs are to make infusions and teas. They're simple to make and can help with a lot of common health problems.

For flu and colds:

To make elderberry tea, mix 2 cups of water with 1 tablespoon of dried elderberries. Bring it to a boil, then let it cook on low for 15 minutes. Strain and drink. Elderberries are famous for making your defense system stronger.

For ginger and lemon tea, cut up a fresh piece of ginger and squeeze some lemon juice into hot water. Let it cook for 10 minutes. This tea is great for easing stuffy noses and sore throats.

For problems with digestion:

For peppermint tea, put 10 minutes' worth of hot water over 1 teaspoon of dried peppermint leaves. When you have trouble digesting food, this tea can help.

For chamomile tea, put 1 teaspoon of dried chamomile flowers in hot water and let them steep for 10 minutes. Chamomile is known to help the digestive system feel better.

To deal with stress and worry:

For Lavender and Lemon Balm Tea, mix dried lavender and lemon balm in equal parts. For 10 minutes, let 1 teaspoon of the mix sit in hot water. This mix helps you relax and feel less stressed.

To make passionflower tea, put a teaspoon of dried passionflower in hot water and let it steep for 10 minutes. Passionflower can help you feel less anxious and sleep better.

Making Your Blends Your Own

When you make your own herbal tea blends, you can change the remedies to fit your wants and tastes. Here are some ways to mix your own teas:

Balance the Flavors: Mix flowers whose flavors go well together. For example, you could mix the sweet licorice root with the hot ginger.

Purposeful Blending: Pick herbs that work on the same illness. For example, to make a strong stomach tea, mix peppermint (which helps digestion) with fennel (which helps with gas).

Try different things: Don't be afraid to try out different amounts and mixtures to see what works best for you.

Essential oils and tinctures
How to Get Ready Step by Step

Herbs that have been soaked in alcohol or vinegar to make tinctures are concentrated versions of those herbs. They are strong and can be kept for a long time. How to make them:

Pick Out Your Herb: Pick either fresh or dried flowers. You should chop fresh herbs very small, but you can use dried herbs as they are.

Fill a Jar: Put half of your choice herb into a glass jar.

Fill the jar all the way to the top with vinegar or alcohol. If you want to use alcohol, choose vodka or brandy. To make tinctures with alcohol, you need to use at least 40% (80 proof) alcohol.

Close the lid tightly on top of the jar and give it a good shake. For four to six weeks, keep the jar in a cool, dark place and shake it every day.

Strain and Bottle: After 4 to 6 weeks, pour the liquid into a clean jar or bottle after straining it through cheesecloth or a fine mesh strainer. Throw away the herbs. Take the medicine and put it in a dark glass bottle. Write the name and date on the bottle.

Instructions for Use and Dosage

Because tinctures are strong, it's important to use them the right way:

In general, one to two dropperfuls (about 30 to 60 drops) should be mixed with water or juice and taken one to three times a day.

Specific Ails: The dose should be followed based on the herb being used and the illness being treated. For instance, echinacea extract might be taken more often when a cold starts to help the immune system.

Using salves and balms to make topical treatments

Herbal oils and beeswax are mixed together to make salves and creams, which are applied to the skin. They are great for easing skin problems and small wounds. Here is a simple recipe:

Add Herbs to Your Oil: Put dried calendula or comfrey in a jar and cover it with a carrier oil like coconut or olive oil. Let it sit for four to six weeks and shake it every day. To speed up the process, you can also slowly heat the jar in a double pot for a few hours.

Strain the Oil: Using cheesecloth, pour the herb-infused oil into a clean jar.

Add Beeswax: Add 1 ounce of beeswax for every cup of blended oil. Use a double pot to melt them both together.

When you're done, pour the mixture into tins or jars and let it cool down.

How to Store and Use Things

Keep salves and balms in cool, dark places to make them last longer, usually up to a year.

How to Use: Put a little on the hurt area and massage it in slowly. As needed to feel better.

How to Make Essential Oil Blends for Different Purposes

Essential oils are strong and can be used in many ways. Here are some basic mixes that you can use every day:

Blend for Relaxation:

Five drops of pure lavender oil

3. Three drops of bergamot oil

2 drops of pure ylang-ylang oil

For a relaxing massage, add to a diffuser or mix with a carrier oil.

Blend for Immune Support:

4 drops of oil from eucalyptus

4. A few drops of tea tree oil

Two drops of pure lemon oil

You can diffuse it in your home or mix it with a carrier oil and rub it on your chest.

Blend for Headaches:

4 drops of pure peppermint oil

Four drops of pure lavender oil

2 drops of pure frankincense oil

Use a carrier oil to thin it out and put it on your temples and the back of your neck.

Safety Rules and How to Dilute

Essential oils are very strong, so be careful when you use them:

Dilution: Before putting essential oils on your skin, you should always mix them with a carrier oil. Two to three drops of essential oil mixed with one teaspoon of neutral oil is a safe amount.

Patch Test: Before using a new essential oil blend, do a patch test to make sure you don't have an allergic response. Place a small amount on your arm and wait 24 hours.

Some essential oils can make people sensitive, or they should not be used in certain situations, like when they are pregnant or with young children. Before using, you should always do some study or talk to an expert.

CHAPTER 5

Remedies for Common Ailments

Colds and Flu
Teas and syrups made from herbs

When it comes to fighting colds and flu, nature is full of herbs that can help ease your symptoms and make your immune system stronger. You can make these plant teas and syrups at home that work well:
Herbal Teas

Blackberry Tea

Two cups of water and one tablespoon of dried elderberries.

To make it, boil water, add elderberries that have been dried, and let it cook for 15 minutes. Strain it and serve it hot.

Elderberries have a lot of antioxidants and vitamins that make your immune system stronger, lower inflammation, and may help shorten the length of colds and flu.

A tea with ginger and lemon

Fresh ginger (one inch cube), lemon, two cups of water, and honey (optional).

Step 1: Cut the ginger into thin slices and add them to water that is heating. Let it cook for 10 minutes. Add honey to taste and squeeze the juice of one lemon into the tea. Drink it hot.

Benefits: Ginger is known to help soothe a sore throat and clear up stuffy noses because it reduces inflammation and viruses. Lemons have vitamin C, which helps your defense system work better.

A tea with chamomile and echinacea

Two cups of water, one teaspoon of dried chamomile leaves, and one teaspoon of dried echinacea.

To make it, boil water, add echinacea and chamomile, and let them soak for 10 minutes. Strain it and serve it hot.

Benefits: Chamomile calms the mind and body, which makes it easier to sleep, and echinacea is known to boost the defense system.

Herbal Syrups

Elderberry syrup

One cup of dried elderberries, four cups of water, and one cup of raw honey.

Elderberries and water should be put in a pot and brought to a boil. Turn down the heat and let it simmer for 45 minutes, or until half of the juice is gone. Strain the mix and let it cool down until it's just warm. Add the honey and mix it in well. You can keep it in the fridge for up to 3 months in a glass jar.

As a regular immune booster, take one tablespoon. During a cold or flu, take one tablespoon every two to three hours.

This syrup is full of immune-boosting chemicals and antioxidants that can help make colds and flu less severe and last shorter.

Honey and ginger syrup

One cup of fresh ginger, two cups of water, one cup of honey, and one lemon's juice.

To get ready, peel and cut the ginger. Put it in a pot with water and heat it up. Let it cook for 30 minutes. Strain it and let it cool down a bit. Mix well after adding the honey and lemon juice. Put it in a glass jar and put it in the fridge for up to one month.

When you have a sore throat or cough, take one teaspoon of this medicine two to three times a day.

Ginger's anti-inflammatory properties and honey's healing properties make this syrup great for getting rid of coughs and sore throats.

Breathing in steam

During a cold or flu, breathing in steam is a great way to clear out your nose and calm down your stuffy lungs. The warmth and wetness help loosen mucus, which makes it easier to cough up. Adding herbs can help even more.
How to Breathe in Steam

Four cups of hot water and a towel.

To get ready, put boiling water in a big bowl. Place a towel over your head and over the bowl to keep the steam inside. Take deep breaths for five to ten minutes.

Advantages: The steam opens up the nasal pathways, lowers swelling, and thins mucus, which makes it easier to get rid of.

Taking in herbal steam

Green Tea and Mint Steam

Five drops of peppermint essential oil, five drops of eucalyptus essential oil, and four cups of hot water.

To make it, add the essential oils to water that is already boiling. Put a towel over your head and lean over the bowl. For 5 to 10 minutes, breathe in the steam.

Peppermint oil helps clear out the lungs and clear up congestion, and eucalyptus oil clears out congestion. When used together, they can help a lot with stuffy noses and chests.

Steam with Chamomile and Thyme

Four cups of boiling water, two tablespoons of dried chamomile leaves, and two tablespoons of dried thyme.

To make it, add the dried herbs to water that is already boiling. Put a towel over your head and lean over the bowl. For 5 to 10 minutes, breathe in the steam.

Benefits: Chamomile can reduce inflammation and calm you down, and thyme is known for killing germs. This mix helps to fight infection and reduce swelling in the nasal passageways.

Steam with Lavender and Rosemary

Five drops of lavender essential oil, five drops of rosemary essential oil, and four cups of hot water.

To make it, add the essential oils to water that is already boiling. Put a towel over your head and lean over the bowl. For 5 to 10 minutes, breathe in the steam.

Good for you: lavender is relaxing and can help you sleep better, and rosemary clears out your lungs and reduces congestion.

Digestive Issues
Teas for Feeling Better

Digestive problems can be painful and get in the way of daily life. Herbal teas are a gentle and effective way to help your body digest food better and calm your stomach. Here are some great drinks that can help settle your stomach:
Tea with ginger

It is well known that ginger can help with digestion. It makes your saliva, bile, and stomach juices come out more, which helps your digestion and eases symptoms like gas, sickness, and bloating.

A bit of fresh ginger that is 1 inch long, 2 cups of water, and honey (optional).

To get ready, peel and cut the ginger. When the water starts to boil, add the ginger slices and let it cook for ten to fifteen minutes. If you want, strain it and add honey.

Benefits: This tea can help with nausea, digestion, and reducing swelling in the digestive system.

Tea with Peppermint

A lot of people use peppermint to ease stomach pain. The menthol in it helps relax the muscles in the digestive system because it has antispasmodic properties.

One teaspoon of dried peppermint leaves and one cup of hot water.

To make it, boil water and add the dried peppermint leaves. Let them steep for 10 minutes. Strain it and serve it hot.

Peppermint tea can help ease the pain and discomfort of indigestion, gas, and bloating. It also helps ease the symptoms of irritable bowel syndrome (IBS).

Fizz Tea

Carminative traits explain why fennel seeds are useful. They stop gas from forming in the intestines and help get rid of gas that is already there.

One teaspoon of fennel seeds and one cup of hot water.

To make it, lightly crush the fennel seeds and let them steep in hot water for 10 minutes. Strain and have fun.

Fennel tea can help your digestive system feel better by easing gas and bloating. Also, it can help ease cramps and keep your gut system healthy in general.

Tea with Chamomile

Chamomile is a gentle plant that has been used for hundreds of years to ease stomachaches and calm the mind.

One teaspoon of dried chamomile leaves and one cup of boiling water.

To make it, boil water and add the dried chamomile flowers. Let them steep for 10 minutes. Strain it and serve it hot.

This tea can help with stomach cramps, bloating, and gas. Chamomile can also help calm you down, which can help with digestive problems caused by worry.

Tonics for digestion

Digestive tonics are made from herbs that help your digestive system stay healthy over time. People usually take them before or after meals to help digestion and avoid stomach pain.
Tonic with apple cider vinegar

Apple cider vinegar (ACV) is a well-known digestive aid that can help keep stomach acid levels in check. This makes it especially helpful for people who don't have enough stomach acid.

One tablespoon of apple cider vinegar, one cup of warm water, and honey, if you want to add it.

To make it, mix the apple cider vinegar with warm water and, if you want, add honey to taste.

To help your body digest food better, drink this tea 15 to 30 minutes before you eat.

Benefits: Apple cider vinegar can help make your stomach more acidic, which can make digestion and nutrient intake better. In addition, it kills germs, which is good for gut health.

Tonic with Lemon and Ginger

This drink has the digestive benefits of ginger and the cleansing effects of lemon.

Lemon juice, a bit of fresh ginger about an inch long, one cup of warm water, and honey (optional).

To make it, grate the ginger and mix it with the warm water and lemon juice. If you want, add honey.

How much to drink: This tonic should be drunk first thing in the morning or before a meal.

Benefits: The lemon helps the body make more bile, which helps digestion, and the ginger makes digestion better and stops feeling sick.

Tonic with Dandelion Root

Dandelion root is a strong gut tonic that can help the liver work better and help the body get rid of toxins.

One teaspoon of dried dandelion root and one cup of hot water.

To make it, boil water and let the dried dandelion root steep for 10 to 15 minutes. Strain and drink.

How much to drink: This tonic should be drunk once or twice a day.

Benefits: Dandelion root helps the body make more bile, which breaks down fat and gets rid of toxins. In addition, it has mild diuretic qualities that can help get rid of gas.

Juice of Aloe Vera

A soothing tonic, aloe vera juice can help with a number of stomach problems, from acid reflux to trouble going to the bathroom.

1/4 cup of pure aloe vera juice and 1 cup of water or natural fruit juice.

To make it, mix the aloe vera juice with water or any fruit drink you like.

To take it, drink 1/4 cup of this mix 20 minutes before you eat.

Benefits: Aloe vera juice can heal and soothe the digestive system, lower inflammation, and help you go to the bathroom regularly.

Skin Conditions
Salve for wounds and cuts that heals

Herbal salves are a great way to heal small cuts and burns. They cover the skin to protect it, lower inflammation, and speed up the mending process. You can make these healing salves at home and they work well:
Salve with Calendula

Calendula is famous for helping skin heal, and it works especially well on cuts, scrapes, and burns.

One cup of calendula-infused oil (made by putting dried calendula flowers into olive oil and letting them steep for a while), one ounce of beeswax, and a few drops of lavender essential oil (optional).

Getting ready:

To make the oil, put dried calendula flowers in a jar and pour olive oil over them. It should sit for 4 to 6 weeks, shaking it every now and then. To speed up the process, you can also heat the jar slowly in a double pot for a few hours.

Strain and Melt: Put the marigold oil into a clean jar after straining it. Melt the beeswax in a double pot, and then add the oil that has calendula in it.

Mix and Pour: Mix the ingredients together until they are well blended. If you want, add a few drops of lavender essential oil. Put it in tins or jars, and then let it cool and harden.

Benefits: Calendula's anti-inflammatory and antimicrobial traits help the body heal faster, lessen pain and swelling, and keep infections from happening.

Salve of Comfrey

Comfrey is another strong herb that can help cuts, scrapes, and small burns heal faster. It has allantoin in it, which helps cells grow and heal.

One cup of comfrey-infused oil (made by letting dried comfrey leaves steep in olive oil for a while), one ounce of beeswax, and ten drops of tea tree essential oil.

Getting ready:

To make the oil, put dried comfrey leaves in a jar and pour olive oil over them. It should sit for 4 to 6 weeks, shaking it every now and then. You can also heat the jar slowly in a double pot for a few hours.

Strain and Melt: Put the comfrey oil through a strainer into a clean jar. Melt the beeswax in a double pot, and then add the oil that has been mixed with comfrey.

Pour and Mix: Mix the ingredients together until they are well blended, then add the tea tree oil. Put it in tins or jars, and then let it cool and harden.

Comfrey helps skin cells heal quickly and reduces inflammation. Tea tree oil, on the other hand, kills germs and keeps infections away.

Plantain Put On

Plantain is a popular weed that can heal you very well. It's great for healing cuts, burns, bug bites, and stings.

One cup of plantain-infused oil (made by putting dried plantain leaves into olive oil and letting them steep for a while), one ounce of beeswax, and ten drops of lavender essential oil.

Getting ready:

To make the oil, put dried plantain leaves in a jar and pour olive oil over them. It should sit for 4 to 6 weeks, shaking it every now and then. You can also heat the jar slowly in a double pot for a few hours.

Strain and Melt: Put the plantain oil into a clean jar after straining it. Melt the beeswax in a double pot, and then add the oil that has been mixed with plantains.

The liquid should be mixed well before it is poured. Add lavender essential oil and stir again. Put it in tins or jars, and then let it cool and harden.

Plantains are good for you because they reduce inflammation and kill germs. Cutting and burning wounds heal faster and with less pain, swelling, and itching.

How to Treat Rash and Irritations

Itching and rashes on the skin can be painful and last for a long time. Using natural remedies to calm the face can help without using harsh chemicals. Ointment with Chamomile

Chamomile is great for healing rashes and irritated skin because it calms and reduces inflammation.

One cup of chamomile-infused oil (made by putting dried chamomile leaves into olive oil and letting them steep for a while), one ounce of beeswax, and ten drops of lavender essential oil.

Getting ready:

To make the oil, put dried chamomile flowers in a jar and pour olive oil over them. It should sit for 4 to 6 weeks, shaking it every now and then. You can also heat the jar slowly in a double pot for a few hours.

Strain and Melt: Put the chamomile oil through a strainer into a clean jar. In a double pot, melt the beeswax. Then, add the oil that has been infused with chamomile.

The liquid should be mixed well before it is poured. Add lavender essential oil and stir again. Put it in tins or jars, and then let it cool and harden.

Advantages: Chamomile salve can lessen the redness, itching, and swelling that come with rashes and other skin problems.

Paste Made of Oats

People know that oatmeal can help with rashes and skin irritations like eczema because it calms and reduces inflammation.

One cup of freshly ground oats and enough water to make a paste.

To make it, mix the ground oats with just enough water to make a thick paste.

How to Use It: Put the paste on the hurt area and let it sit for 15 to 20 minutes. Then, wash it off with cool water.

Benefits: Oatmeal can help soothe skin that is itchy, reduce swelling, and keep it wet.

Green Aloe Gel

Aloe vera can help heal a lot of different skin problems. It works great for easing rashes and skin that is itchy.

Fresh aloe vera leaf is what it's made of.

To get ready, cut open a new aloe vera leaf and take the gel out of the center.

Application: Put the gel on the skin directly where it hurts and let it soak in.

Aloe vera juice can help soothe and heal rashes and skin irritations because it cools, reduces inflammation, and moisturizes the skin.

Stress and Anxiety

Baths and teas that calm you down

Managing worry and anxiety is important for health in general. Herbal teas and baths that calm you down are examples of natural remedies that can help you feel better and sleep.
Teas for Relaxing

Chai tea is an easy way to calm your body and mind that works well. Here are some mixes that are known to help you relax:
Tea with Chamomile

Chamomile is one of the best known herbs for sleep and stress relief.

One teaspoon of dried chamomile leaves, one cup of boiling water, and honey, if you want to add some.

To make it, boil water and add the dried chamomile flowers. Let them steep for 10 minutes. If you want, strain it and add honey.

Chamomile tea can help you feel less stressed, sleep better, and calm down. It's a great way to relax before bed because it has mild calming effects.

Chamomile Tea

Lavender is known for its ability to calm and soothe.

One teaspoon of dried lavender buds, one cup of hot water, and honey, if you want to add it.

To make it, boil water and let the dried lavender buds soak for 5 to 10 minutes. If you want, strain it and add honey.

Lavender tea can help relieve stress and anxiety, get rid of headaches, and make you feel more relaxed. Its soft flower scent also adds to the relaxing effect.

Tea with Lemon Balm

Lemon balm is a type of mint that is known to help calm people down.

One teaspoon of dried lemon balm leaves and one cup of hot water.

To make it, boil water and add the dried lemon balm leaves. Let them steep for 10 minutes. Strain and have fun.

Lemon balm tea can help lower stress, boost your happiness, and help you sleep better. People also know that it can make them feel a little sleepy.

Tea with Passionflower

People often use passionflower to help them sleep and deal with worry.

One teaspoon of dried passionflower and one cup of hot water.

To make it, boil water and let the dried passionflower steep for 10 minutes.
Strain it and serve it hot.

Benefits: Drinking passionflower tea can help you feel less anxious and more calm. It works especially well for treating insomnia caused by worry.

Baths that relax

Taking a warm bath with herbs and essential oils in it can be very relaxing and help ease stress and anxiety.
Tub with Lavender

Lavender is great for a peaceful bath because it calms you down.

You will need 1 cup of Epsom salts, 10 drops of lavender essential oil, and 1/2 cup of dried lavender flowers, but they are not required.

In a bowl, mix Epsom salts and lavender essential oil together. If you want to, add dried lavender flowers. This should be put into a warm bath and left there for at least 20 minutes.

Benefits: Epsom salts and lavender together help to calm you down, relax your muscles, and ease stress. The smell of lavender also helps you sleep.

Bath with Chamomile and Oatmeal

This bath is good for your face and your mind.

One cup of oatmeal, one cup of dried chamomile leaves, and a muslin bag or cheesecloth.

Step 1: Put the oatmeal and dried chamomile flowers in the muslin bag or fabric and tie it up tightly. Put it in the bathwater and let it soak in for a while. Enjoy a 20-minute soak in the tub.

Chamomile can help calm your mind and lower your stress, and oatmeal can soothe and moisturize your skin.

A bath with milk and roses

A luxurious bath that helps you rest and keeps your skin healthy.

One cup of dried rose petals, two cups of milk, and ten drops of rose essential oil.

To make it, heat up a bath and add milk and dried rose petals. Mix the water by adding rose essential oil and stirring it in. Enjoy a 20-minute soak in the tub.

Benefits: Rose petals and essential oil can calm and uplift you, and milk can feed and soften your skin.

Blends for aromatherapy

Essential oils are used in aromatherapy to help people rest and feel less stressed and anxious. You can use these mixes in diffusers, massage oils, or inhalers and they will work well.
Blend for Relaxation

A classic mix that makes you feel calm and at ease.

Five drops of lavender essential oil, three drops of bergamot essential oil, and two drops of ylang-ylang essential oil.

To get ready, put the essential oils in a diffuser with water or mix them with a carrier oil to make a massage more relaxing.

Benefits: This blend is great for making the surroundings calm and stress-free. Bergamot makes you feel better, lavender calms you down, and ylang-ylang makes you feel less anxious.

Blend for Stress Relief

A mix that is meant to ease worry and tension.

It has 2 drops of lemon essential oil, 4 drops of frankincense essential oil, and 4 drops of clary sage essential oil.

To make the mixture, put the essential oils in a burner or mix them with a carrier oil to put on the skin.

Frankincense helps you breathe deeper and calm your mind. Clary sage eases stress and tension, and lemon makes you feel better and more alert.

Blend for Sleepy Time

A mix to help you sleep well and feel less anxious at night.

Five drops of lavender essential oil, three drops of chamomile essential oil, and two drops of cedarwood essential oil.

To get ready, put the essential oils in a diffuser or put them on your pulse points before bed after diluting them in a carrier oil.

Lavender and chamomile help you relax and sleep, and cedarwood can help calm an anxious mind by making you feel grounded.

Blend to Uplift

A mix to improve your mood and calm you down.

Five drops of orange essential oil, three drops of peppermint essential oil, and two drops of geranium essential oil.

To make the massage, either put the essential oils in a diffuser or mix them with a carrier oil.

Orange and peppermint scents make you feel good and give you energy. Geranium, on the other hand, balances your feelings and calms you down.

Minor Injuries and Pain Relief
Topical salves for pain relief

Pain relief salves that you put on the wound are a great way to treat small injuries like scrapes, bruises, and sore muscles. Healing herbs, a carrier oil, and beeswax are often mixed together in these salves to make a soothing balm that is easy to put on the skin.
Salve for Arnica

It is well known that arnica can help lessen pain and inflammation. It works especially well for healing bruises and sore muscles.

One cup of arnica-infused oil (made by putting dried arnica flowers in olive oil and letting them steep), one ounce of beeswax, and ten drops of lavender essential oil.

Getting ready:

To make the oil, put dried arnica flowers in a jar and pour olive oil over them. It should sit for 4 to 6 weeks, shaking it every now and then. You can also heat the jar slowly in a double pot for a few hours.

Step 2: Strain the arnica oil into a clean jar. Do this again to melt it. In a double pot, melt the beeswax. Then, add the oil that has been mixed with arnica.

The liquid should be mixed well before it is poured. Add lavender essential oil and stir again. Put it in tins or jars, and then let it cool and harden.

Advantages: Arnica cream lowers swelling, eases pain, and speeds up the healing process for cuts and bruises.

Salve with Cayenne

Cayenne pepper has a chemical called capsaicin in it that naturally eases pain. It lowers the amount of substance P in the body, which is a chemical that tells the brain about pain.

One cup of cayenne-infused oil (made by adding cayenne pepper to olive oil and letting it steep), one ounce of beeswax, and ten drops of peppermint essential oil.

Getting ready:

Mix the Oil: Put the cayenne pepper in a jar and pour olive oil over it. It should sit for 4 to 6 weeks, shaking it every now and then. You can also heat the jar slowly in a double pot for a few hours.

Strain and Melt: Put the chili oil into a clean jar after straining it. Melt the beeswax in a double pot, and then add the oil that has been mixed with cayenne.

Pour and Mix: Mix the ingredients together, then add the peppermint essential oil. Put it in tins or jars, and then let it cool and harden.

Advantages: Cayenne balm eases pain in muscles and joints, lowers swelling, and boosts blood flow.

Salve of St. John's Wort

People know that St. John's Wort can ease pain and reduce inflammation. This medicine works especially well for nerve pain and small cuts.

One cup of oil made by putting dried St. John's Wort into olive oil and letting it steep for a while, one ounce of beeswax, and ten drops of tea tree essential oil.

Getting ready:

Put the dried St. John's Wort in a jar and top it with olive oil. It should sit for 4 to 6 weeks, shaking it every now and then. You can also heat the jar slowly in a double pot for a few hours.

Strain and Melt: Put the St. John's Wort oil through a strainer into a clean jar. In a double pot, melt the beeswax. Then, add the oil that has St. John's Wort in it.

Pour and Mix: Mix the ingredients together until they are well blended, then add the tea tree oil. Put it in tins or jars, and then let it cool and harden.

Benefits: St. John's Wort salve eases nerve pain, lowers swelling, and speeds up the healing of small cuts and scrapes.

Herbal Tinctures for Pain Relief

Herbal medicines are concentrated extracts of plants that can be taken by mouth to ease pain. They work well for a wide range of pain situations because they are strong.
Tincture of Willow Bark

Willow bark has been used to treat pain naturally for hundreds of years. It has salicin in it, which is changed by the body into salicylic acid, which is like aspirin.

Two cups of vodka (or another strong booze) and one cup of dried willow bark.

Getting ready:

Fill a Jar: Put the dried willow wood into a glass jar.

Liquor: Fill the jar all the way up with vodka and pour it over the willow leaves.

Close the lid tightly on top of the jar and give it a good shake. For four to six weeks, keep the jar in a cool, dark place and shake it every day.

Put the juice through a cheesecloth and into a clean jar or bottle. This should be done after 4 to 6 weeks. Throw away the willow bark. Take the medicine and put it in a dark glass bottle. Write the name and date on the bottle.

To use, mix one to two dropperfuls (about 30 to 60 drops) with water or juice and take it up to three times a day.

Benefits: Headaches, joint pain, and arthritis can all be helped by willow bark tincture.

A mixture of turmeric and ginger

Both turmeric and ginger are very good at reducing inflammation, which means that this liquid can help with pain.

1/2 cup of dried ginger root, 1/2 cup of dried turmeric root, and 2 cups of vodka (or another strong booze).

Getting ready:

Fill a Jar: Put the dried ginger root and turmeric in a glass jar.

Place the leaves in a jar and fill it up with vodka until it's full.

Close the lid tightly on top of the jar and give it a good shake. For four to six weeks, keep the jar in a cool, dark place and shake it every day.

Put the juice through a cheesecloth and into a clean jar or bottle. This should be done after 4 to 6 weeks. Throw away the herbs. Take the medicine and put it in a dark glass bottle. Write the name and date on the bottle.

To use, mix one to two dropperfuls (about 30 to 60 drops) with water or juice and take it up to three times a day.

Benefits: This liquid lowers swelling, eases joint pain, and boosts the immune system as a whole.

Tincture of Valerian Root

Valerian root is known to calm people down and relax muscles, which makes it great for relieving pain and helping people sleep well.

Two cups of vodka (or another high-proof booze) and one cup of dried valerian root.

Getting ready:

Put the dried valerian root in a glass jar to fill it up.

Put in some alcohol. Fill the jar all the way up with vodka poured over the valerian root.

Close the lid tightly on top of the jar and give it a good shake. For four to six weeks, keep the jar in a cool, dark place and shake it every day.

Put the juice through a cheesecloth and into a clean jar or bottle. This should be done after 4 to 6 weeks. Throw away the valerian root. Take the medicine and put it in a dark glass bottle. Write the name and date on the bottle.

Dosage: Mix one to two dropperfuls (about 30 to 60 drops) with water or drink and take it up to three times a day, preferably before bed.

Valerian root medicine can help relax muscles, ease pain, and help you sleep well.

THE END

www.ingramcontent.com/pod-product-compliance
Lightning Source LLC
LaVergne TN
LVHW022315070125
800770LV00029B/1021